Over 750,000 people in the U.S. have some type of ostomy. Most have the same type that you have—a colostomy.

Having a colostomy can be scary at first. It may be hard to get used to, but a colostomy is not a handicap. In fact, your colostomy will help you live a longer, healthier, more active life.

The sooner you learn how to care for your colostomy, the better you will feel about yourself.

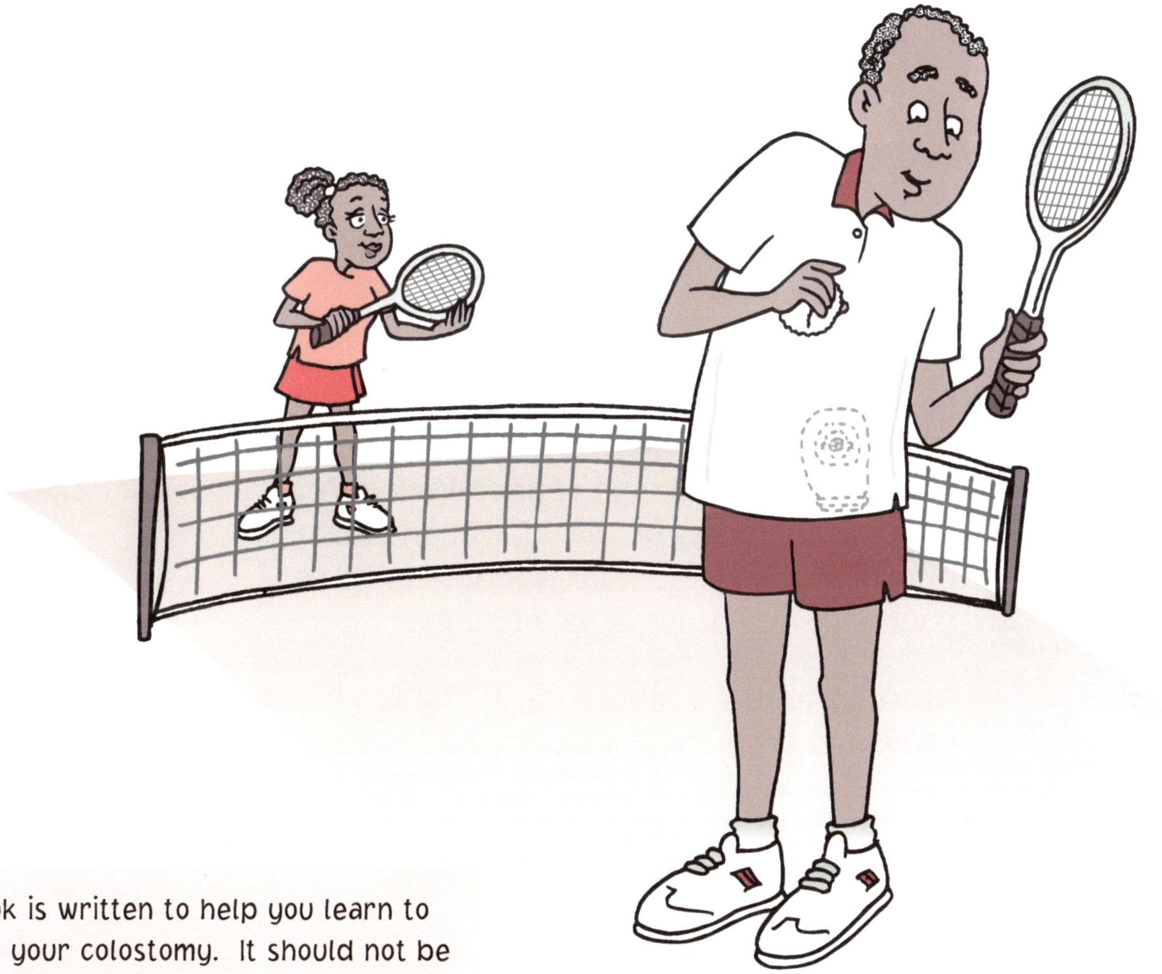

This book is written to help you learn to care for your colostomy. It should not be used to replace any treatment or advice from your doctor or WOC (Wound, Ostomy, Continence) nurse.

Definitions

Clamp – a plastic closure that is placed on the end of a drainable pouch to allow you to empty the pouch.

Colostomy – the end of the colon that opens on your abdomen and lets the stool out.

Ostomy – another word for stoma.

Pouch – the plastic bag that collects stool. It has a skin barrier wafer that protects the skin around the stoma. Pouches are clear or opaque and are odor-proof.

Skin Barrier – the part of the pouch that sticks to the skin. It is usually a gold or brown color.

Skin Sealant – a wipe or spray that puts a clear coating on the skin to protect it from irritation caused by urine, stool or tape. It can also be used to seal stoma powders in when treating irritated skin.

Stoma – the opening in your abdomen from your colon. It may be raised, wet and deep pink or red in color. It allows stool to leave your body. It has no nerve endings.

Stoma Paste – a special paste that works like caulking to seal the pouch around the stoma.

Stoma Powder – a special powder used to treat irritated skin around the stoma.

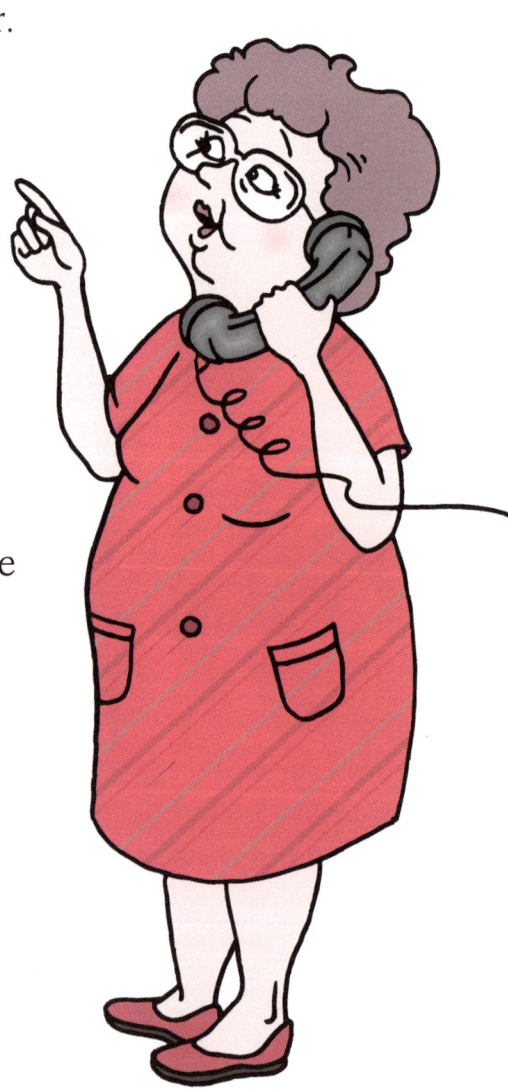

How digestion works

When you eat, food goes from your esophagus (food pipe) into your stomach. In the stomach, food is changed into a liquid. Then the liquid goes to your small intestine. All digestion of food takes place in your small intestine.

The small intestine absorbs (takes in) what the body needs. Any undigested food (waste), water and stomach juices (enzymes) then pass into the colon. The colon stores the stool and absorbs water from your stool. As waste matter passes along the colon, the liquid is absorbed from it, and stool becomes firmer. Stool is stored in your colon until you have a bowel movement.

Surgery is done when the large intestine can no longer handle waste matter going through it. The stool is "re-routed" around the diseased area of the colon. To do this, a surgical opening in your colon, called a colostomy is made.

There is no sphincter muscle with a colostomy, so you cannot control or hold back stool as it leaves your body.

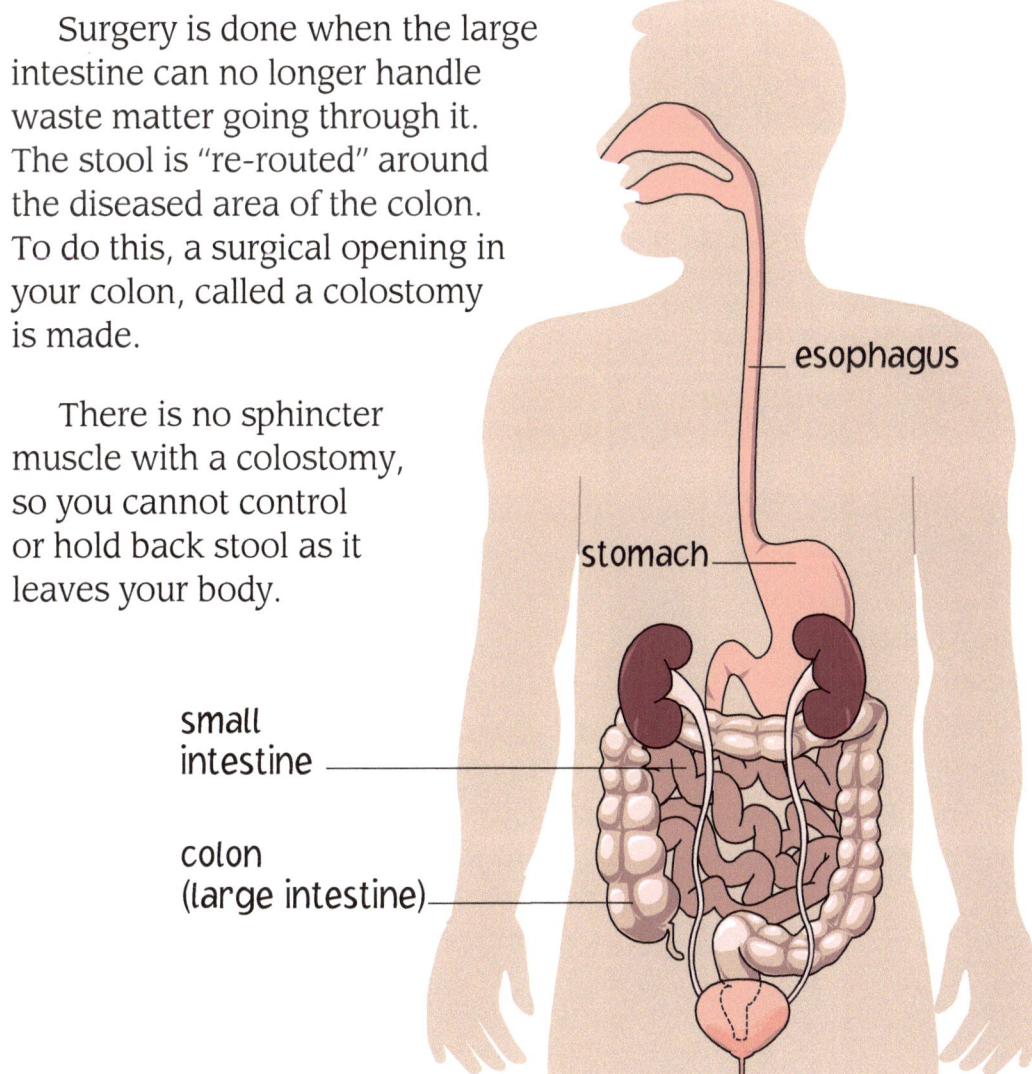

esophagus

stomach

small intestine

colon (large intestine)

The operation

During colostomy surgery, the doctor cuts the colon into two pieces. One end of the colon is sewn into an opening made in the abdominal wall. The rest of the colon is removed or bypassed. A colostomy is permanent if your sphincter muscle is removed. A colostomy can also be temporary if part of your colon is only bypassed until it heals.

There are 4 types of colostomies:

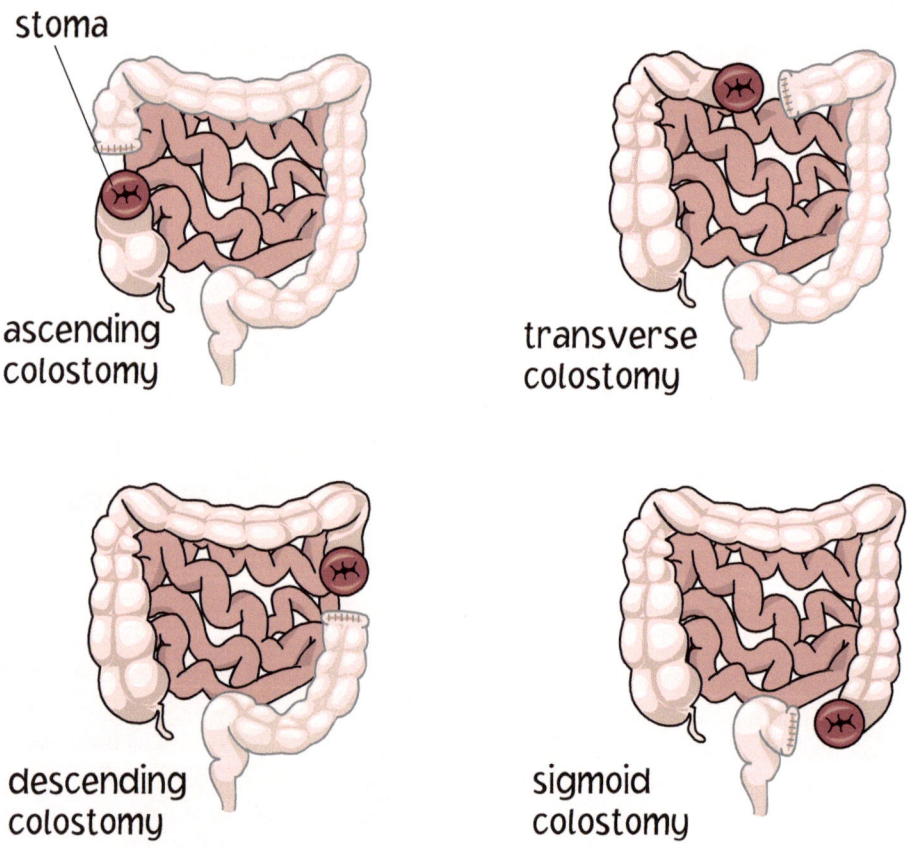

stoma

ascending colostomy

transverse colostomy

descending colostomy

sigmoid colostomy

The firmness of stool from each type of colostomy is different. As waste moves through the colon, water is absorbed from it and the stool becomes more solid. Stool from an ascending colostomy is still liquid, but stool from a sigmoid colostomy is like normal stool.

You have a _____ colostomy, so your

stool will likely be _____.

Your stoma

The opening on your abdomen is called a "stoma" or ostomy. Intestines have no nerves, so the stoma will not hurt. But intestines do have a lot of blood vessels. This means your stoma will be wet and deep pink or red in color and may bleed a little when it is touched or rubbed.

After surgery, your stoma will be swollen. It will get smaller over 6–8 weeks. After that, most stomas remain the same size unless you lose or gain weight.

With a colostomy you wear a pouch which collects stool and protects the skin around your stoma. The opening in the pouch should fit close to your stoma (about $\frac{1}{8}''$) without a lot of skin showing when the pouch is on.

To find the right stoma opening size for your pouch, measure the base of your stoma. Your WOC nurse will show you how.

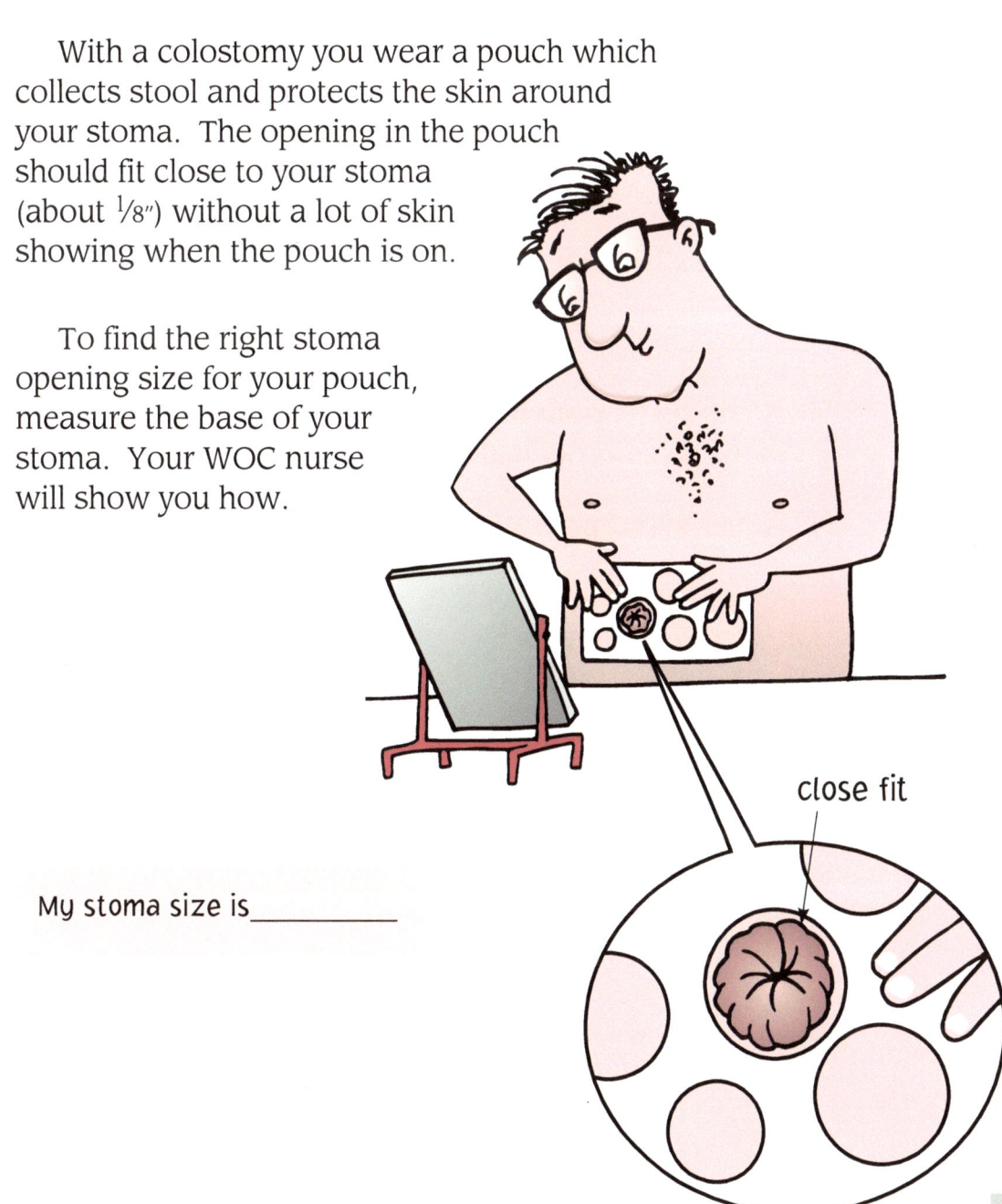

close fit

My stoma size is_____

Colostomy pouches

A pouch is a clear or opaque, odor-proof bag. A special skin barrier wafer sticks it to the skin. There are different types of pouches. There are 1-piece, 2-piece, drainable, closed-end, cut-to-fit and pre-sized pouches.

- **A 1-piece pouch** has a skin barrier wafer attached to the pouch that sticks to the skin.

- **A 2-piece pouch** has a skin barrier wafer or flange that sticks to the skin and a pouch that snaps on or off of the wafer or flange.

- **A drainable pouch** can be opened at the bottom so stool can be emptied out. It is then closed with a pouch clamp.

- **A closed-end pouch** has no opening at the bottom so stool cannot be emptied out. There is no clamp.

- **A cut-to-fit pouch** allows you to cut the opening in the skin barrier wafer to fit your stoma.

- **A pre-sized pouch** is ordered for the size of your stoma and does not need to be cut.

Ask your WOC nurse which pouch is right for you.

If your pouch doesn't fit well, it may leak or allow odor to escape. This is a special concern for people who have ascending and transverse colostomies. Stool from these stomas has digestive juices (enzymes) that can hurt your skin. Itching or burning under your pouch may mean you have a leak. It is very important to have a good fit.

The best pouch for me is a _____ pouch.

Emptying a drainable pouch

Empty your pouch when it is ⅓ to ½ full of stool or has begun to fill with gas.

1. Sit on the toilet, in front of it or next to it – whatever is easiest for you. Remove the clamp and fold back (cuff) the bottom of the pouch.

2. Point the bottom of your pouch into the toilet. Let the stool drain into the toilet.

3. Clean the tail end of the pouch with toilet paper or a baby wipe.

4. If you are concerned about odors, put mouthwash or deodorant into the pouch.

5. Uncuff the bottom of the pouch, close and clamp it. Make sure it is sealed.

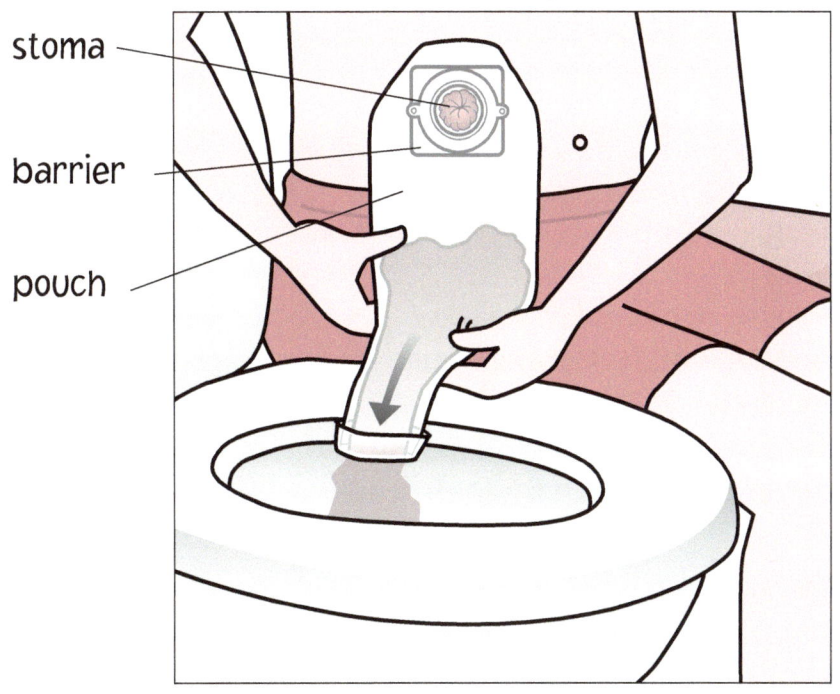

stoma

barrier

pouch

Changing a 1-piece pouch

How often you change your pouch depends on the type of skin barrier wafer you have. It also depends on your personal choice. Some barriers can last as long as 14 days. But you may want to change it on a regular schedule (every Sunday, for example). Change it right away if your skin begins to burn, itch or if your pouch leaks.

The best time to change your pouch is before you eat or drink anything each

1. First get all supplies ready. Check what you need:

❑ a pouch

❑ a pattern for your stoma

❑ scissors
    (if cutting your barrier)

❑ warm water

❑ soft cloths or paper towels

❑ skin sealant

❑ stoma paste (if using it)

❑ a plastic trash bag

❑ other_____

    _____

2. Empty your old pouch.

3. Take off the used pouch by gently lifting any tape around the skin barrier. Be careful not to hurt your skin.

4. Use one hand to hold the pouch. With your other hand, use a damp cloth to gently push your skin away from where the pouch is stuck. Save the clamp for later.

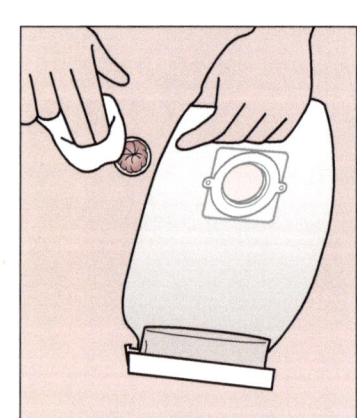

5. Put the old pouch in the plastic bag.

6. Gently wash your skin and stoma with a soft cloth or paper towel and warm water. When you are finished, put the throw away items in the plastic bag.

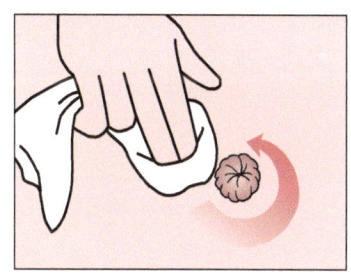

7. Check your stoma. Note any change in size or color, any cuts or unusual bleeding. You may see a small amount of bleeding when you clean your stoma. This is OK.

8. Get your new pouch ready. If you cut the skin barrier wafer, cut it using the right sized pattern for your stoma. If you use a pre-sized pouch, take off the paper backing. Put the pouch aside.

9. Check the skin around your stoma for any redness or rash. See page 14 for how to treat skin irritation.

10. Make sure your skin is dry so the skin barrier will stick to your skin. Center and press the new barrier/pouch against the skin around your stoma. Make sure the barrier feels OK. Put the clamp on.

barrier   tape

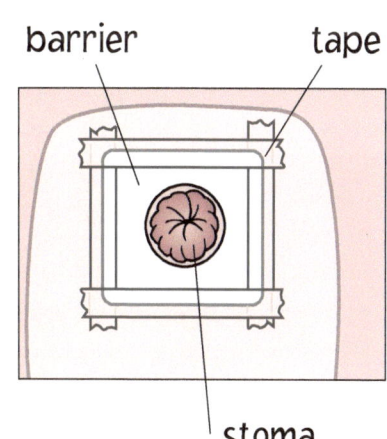

stoma

11. If you use tape around the barrier, be sure to use skin sealant first and let it dry. Then tape as you were taught.

12. Put all other throw away items in the plastic bag and throw it away.

If you have trouble with your pouch leaking or not sticking well, talk with your WOC nurse about using stoma

Changing a 2-Piece Pouch

A 2-piece pouch has a skin barrier wafer or flange and a snap on pouch. You can change your pouch every day or when you like. How often you change your flange depends on the type of barrier you have and your personal choice. Some flanges can stay on as long as 14 days. You may want to change the barrier on a regular schedule, like every Sunday. Change it right away if your skin begins to burn, itch or if your pouch leaks.

1. First, get all supplies ready. Check what you need:

Change your pouch before you eat or drink

❏ pouch and barrier

❏ a pattern and scissors (if cutting the flange)

❏ a plastic trash bag

❏ warm water

❏ stoma paste (if you use it)

❏ skin sealant

❏ soft wash cloths or paper towels

❏ other_____

2. Empty your old pouch.

3. Take off the used flange and pouch by gently lifting any tape around the flange. Be careful not to hurt your skin. Save the clamp for later.

4. Use one hand to hold the flange. With the other hand, use a damp cloth or paper towel to gently push your skin away from where the flange is stuck.

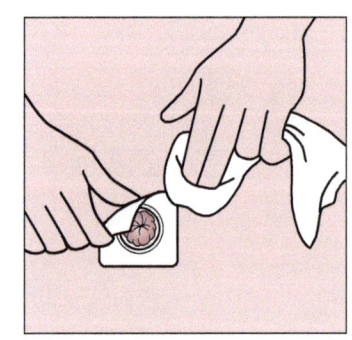

5. Put the used flange in the plastic bag. (If you can reuse your pouch, see page 12 for how to clean it.)

If you have trouble with your pouch leaking or not sticking well, talk with your WOC nurse about what you can do to get a better

6. Gently wash your skin and stoma with a soft cloth or paper towel and warm water. When you are finished, put the throw away items in the plastic bag.

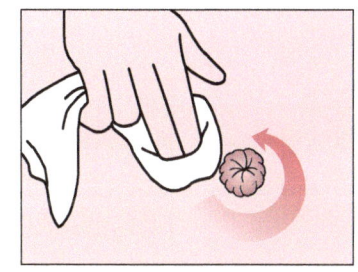

7. Check your stoma. Note any change in size or color, any cuts or unusual bleeding. You may see a small amount of bleeding when you clean your stoma. This is OK.

8. Get your new flange ready. If you cut it out, measure your stoma and cut the flange using the correct sized pattern. Remove the paper from the back of the new flange.

9. Check the skin around your stoma for redness or rash.

10. Be sure your skin is dry. Center the new flange over your stoma and press it to your skin. Snap the pouch on the flange. Put the clamp on.

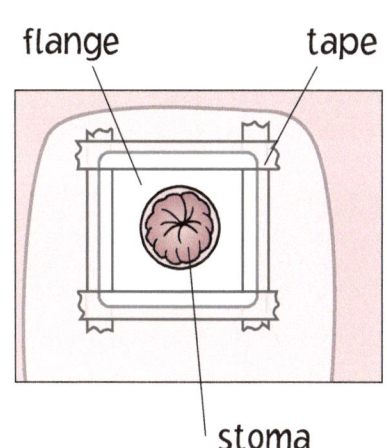

flange   tape

stoma

11. If you use tape around the flange, be sure to use skin sealant first and let it dry. Then tape as you were taught.

12. Put all other throw away items in the plastic bag, tie it off and throw it away.

Even though pouches are odor-proof, you may want to use a deodorizer in your pouch or take a special pill to help prevent odor. Ask your WOC nurse about

Cleaning your 2-piece pouch

If you plan to use your pouch again, follow these steps to clean it:

1. Get two 1-quart squirt or spray bottles.

2. Put cool water in one bottle. Add about ¼ to ½ teaspoon of any kind of liquid soap. Mix well.

3. Put cool water in the other bottle and add 10-12 drops of any kind of liquid fabric softener.

4. Hold the used pouch over the toilet. Spray or squirt with the soapy water. Rub until clean. Empty into toilet.

5. Hold the pouch over the toilet and rinse with the fabric softener water. Empty into toilet. This will keep the plastic soft and smelling fresh.

6. Hang the pouch up to air dry.

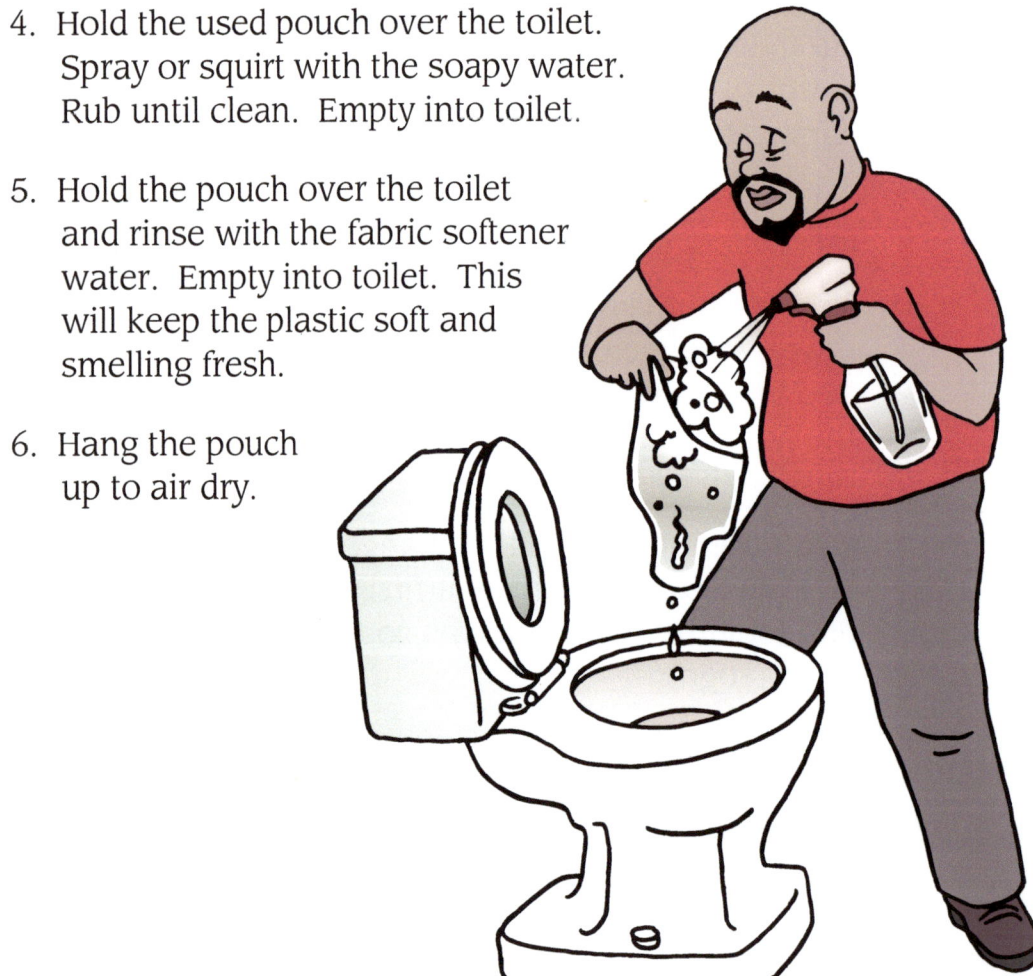

tips for pouch care

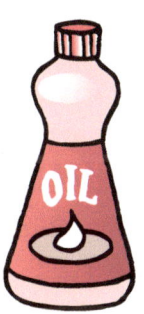

- To make emptying easier, use ½ teaspoon mineral oil, or spray a little cooking oil into the pouch after you clean it and before you put it back on.

- Before emptying, place some toilet paper in the bowl to avoid splashing.

- Leave a little air inside your pouch to keep it from sticking to your moist stoma.

- When you apply a new pouch, angle it slightly toward your groin to make emptying easier. This works well if you sit on the toilet to empty.

- Ask your WOC nurse how many times you can use each pouch.

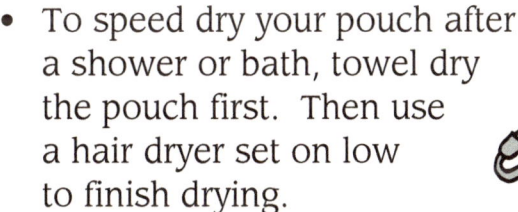

- To speed dry your pouch after a shower or bath, towel dry the pouch first. Then use a hair dryer set on low to finish drying.

- With both 1-piece and 2-piece drainable types of pouches, you need to clean the bottom inch of the pouch and/or cuff well. If this area is not cleaned well, odor may occur and stool could get on your underclothes.

Ask your WOC nurse for help
if your pouch isn't staying on
or if your skin stays irritated.

Peristomal (pear-ee-stomal) skin care

The peristomal skin (the skin around your stoma) must stay clean and healthy. **Each time you change your pouch, check the stoma and skin around it for signs of infection or irritation**. These include changes in the color or size of stoma or the skin around it feeling warm to the touch. If you have any of these signs:

1. Apply skin barrier powder if the skin is irritated and if your WOC nurse said it is OK. Seal in the powder with a skin sealant in "wipe-on" or spray form, or wet your finger with water to apply. A skin sealant also protects the skin around the stoma from tape.

   Skin sealants in "wipe-on" form come with and without alcohol. It's OK to use a skin sealant with alcohol when your skin is clear or only a little red. When your skin is raw or very red use the skin sealant without alcohol to avoid burning.

2. Repeat these steps (powder then sealant) 1 or 2 times to form a crust if the skin is raw. Make sure the last layer is a sealant—not a powder. Once the crust is dry, apply your pouch barrier. You can use a hair dryer on a low or cool setting to dry your skin.

3. Call your WOC nurse if your skin has not improved the next time you change your pouch. Your nurse may want you to use some other treatment for skin problems.

What to Report

Call your doctor or WOC nurse if you have any of these:

- **cramps** lasting more than **2 to 3 hours**

- new **red or irritated areas of skin around** your **stoma**

- **signs of infection** around the stoma: **red, weepy skin** that is **warm to the touch**

- **fever** above 101°F (38.3°C) by mouth

- **drainage from incision area**

- **severe constipation** or **diarrhea**

- **nausea** or **vomiting** that **won't stop**

- **a steady leaking of blood** from your stoma for 2-3 hours or more

- **a sudden gush of blood** of 1-2 tablespoons or more

Also, **watch for other changes in your stool**. Tell your doctor or WOC nurse if it is **more watery, a different color or bloody**.

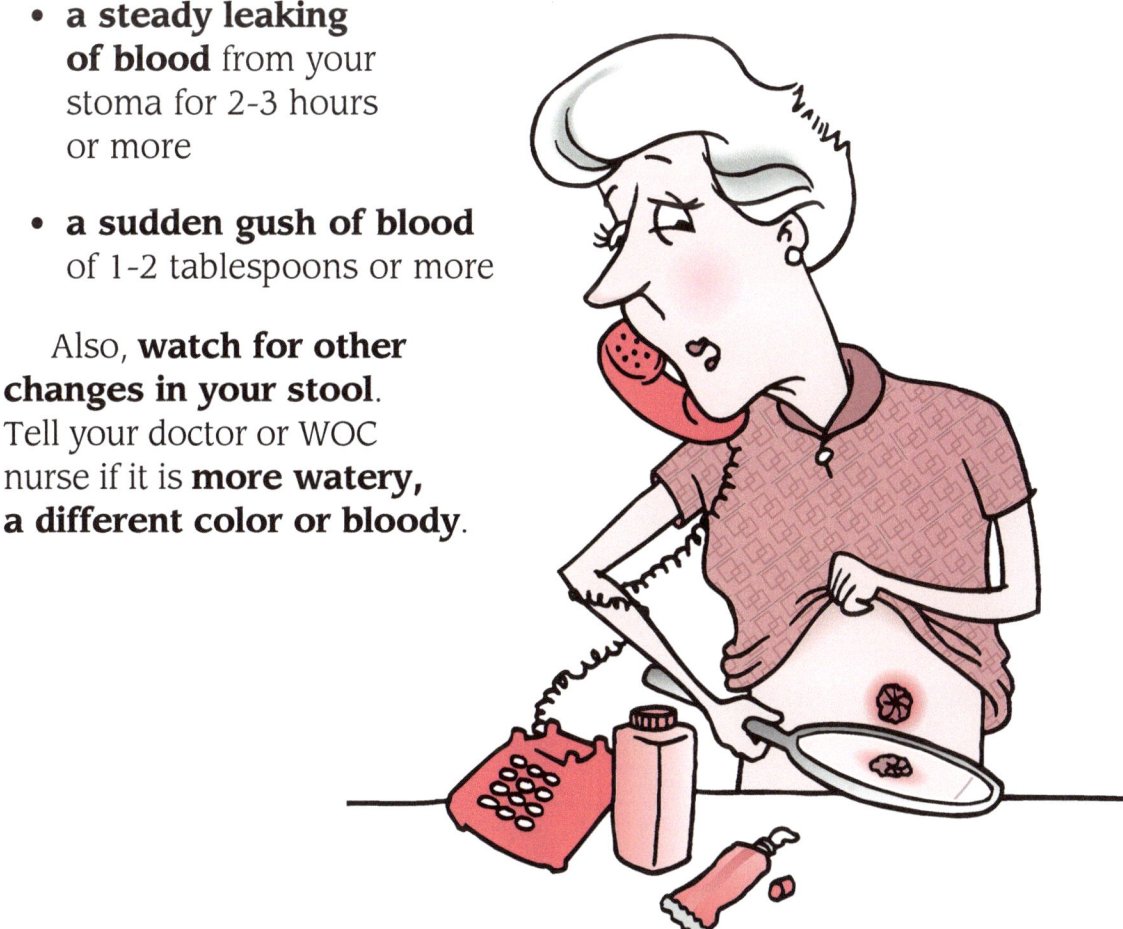

Irrigation

Some people with descending or sigmoid colostomies can have more control of their bowel movements by irrigating. **Irrigation** is an enema through the stoma. It **trains the colon to empty at a regular time** each day or every other day. In many cases, irrigation lets a person with a colostomy go without a pouch and just wear a small stoma cap or use a closed-end or security pouch. Closed-end pouches come as a 1-piece system or a 2-piece system. Some of these pouches also have a charcoal gas filter to release gas without causing odor.

   Do not try to irrigate without talking to your doctor or WOC nurse first.

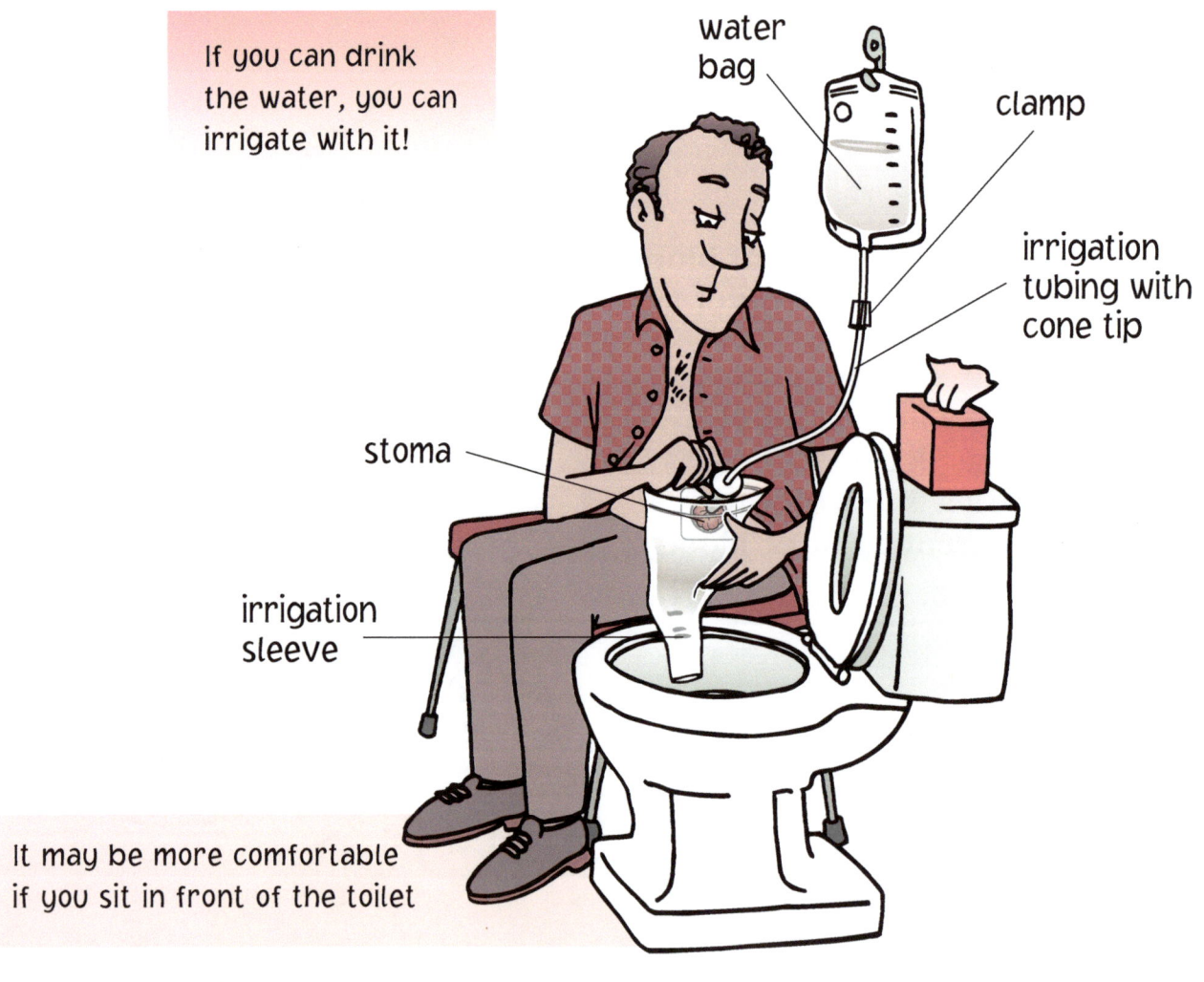

If you can drink the water, you can irrigate with it!

water bag

clamp

irrigation tubing with cone tip

stoma

irrigation sleeve

It may be more comfortable if you sit in front of the toilet

How to irrigate

Irrigate every day, every other day, or as your doctor or WOC nurse tells you. Irrigation will start a bowel movement. It is best to try to irrigate about the same time each day.

1. Clamp the irrigation tubing, then fill your water bag with about 1 quart of warm water. (Cold water can cause cramps and hot water can damage your bowel.) The bottom of the bag should be level with your shoulder. This is to avoid cramps. Hang the bag on a hook or nail.

2. Remove your pouch, and put on an irrigation sleeve without the clamp. Hang the end of the irrigation sleeve in the toilet.

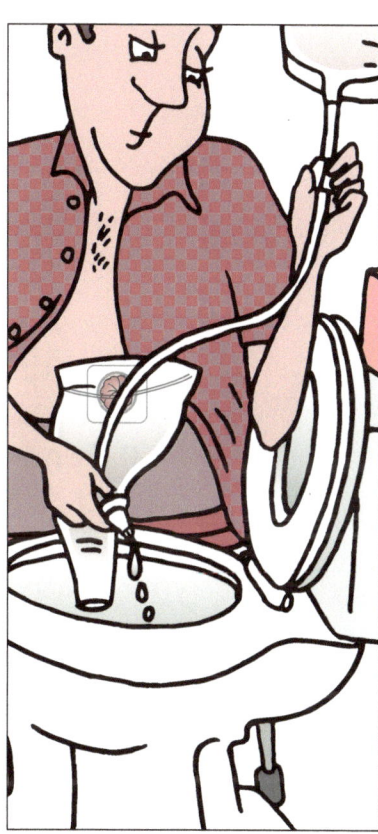

3. Release the clamp on the irrigation bag. Flush the tubing with water until the water starts coming out of the cone tip. This will help stop air from getting into your colon (which can cause cramps). Reclamp the tube.

4. Lubricate the cone tip with K-Y® or any water soluble lubricant (not Vaseline®) and gently push the cone into your stoma.

5. Release the clamp on the tubing to start the flow of water. The water should go in slowly over 5–8 minutes. Remove the cone when the water is in.

6. If you get cramps, don't take the cone out. Clamp the tube and wait until the cramps go away. Then unclamp the tube and let the rest of the water flow in.

7. Part of the water and stool will come back out of your stoma right away. Most of the water and stool will come out about 15–30 minutes later.

8. After waiting about 5-10 minutes, you can lift the sleeve out of the toilet and dry the end. Fold up the end of the sleeve, and clamp it shut until the rest of the stool and water are collected. Do this so you can move around while waiting for your colon to empty.

9. Return to the bathroom in 20–30 minutes to clean the sleeve and put on a clean pouch as you have been taught.

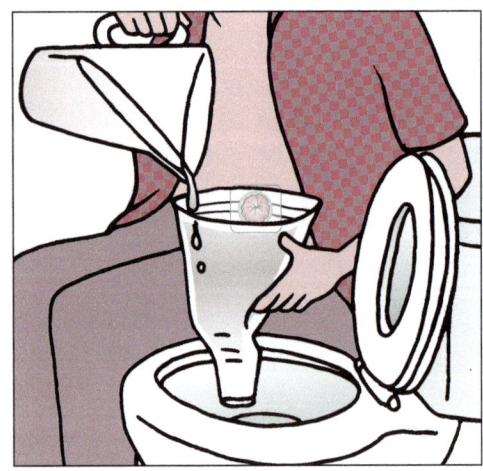

Tip: Keep a pitcher of water near the toilet to rinse the sleeve before you take it

Diet

With a colostomy, you should **avoid spicy or greasy foods for the first 4–6 weeks after your surgery**. Then try new foods one at a time to see how your body handles them. Try just a little of each new food and see what happens (1-2 tablespoons is best).

As a rule, once you have healed you can return to a normal diet, unless you are already on a special diet. You should **make sure to get enough fluids.** Eat foods that have **potassium** in them* (unless your doctor tells you not to). You need a good balance of all these nutrients to stay healthy.

When you have a colostomy, gas can be a problem. It can make your ostomy pouch bulge. To keep from getting gas:

- eat slowly and **chew your food well**

- **limit** the amount of **foods that give you gas**

- **eat** your meals at **about the same times each day**

- **avoid skipping meals**

- **limit dairy products**, especially if you are lactose intolerant

- **sip** liquids **slowly**

- **avoid chewing gum, straws** and **talking while eating**

- **limit carbonated drinks** (like sodas and beer)

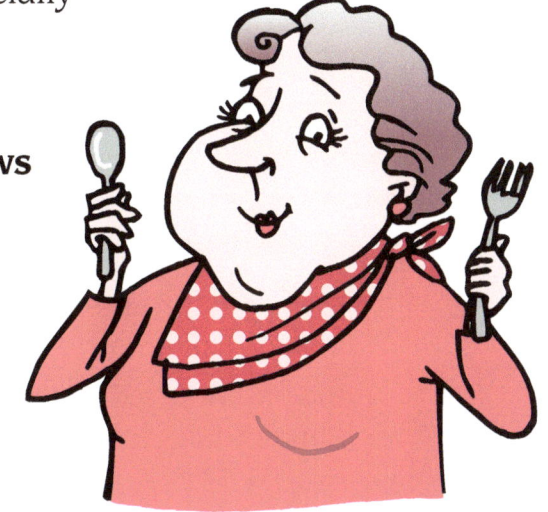

* Raisins, strawberries, bananas, oranges, beans,

Choose your foods wisely, and notice how different foods affect your body. These lists will help you in your food choices.

Foods that may cause gas

- beans
- beer
- broccoli
- cabbage
- cauliflower
- cheese
- corn
- garlic
- milk
- onions
- sodas

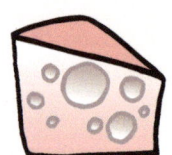

Foods that caused you gas and odor before surgery will most likely do the same after surgery.

Foods that may thicken your stool

- applesauce
- bananas
- buttermilk
- cheese
- marshmallows
- milk (boiled)
- noodles
- peanut butter creamy, not chunky)
- pretzels
- rice
- toast
- yogurt
- pudding

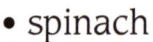
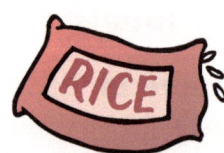

These foods may help if you get diarrhea.

Foods that may loosen your stool

- beer
- broccoli
- grape juice
- fresh fruits (except bananas)
- green beans
- prunes or prune juice
- spicy foods

- spinach
- fried foods

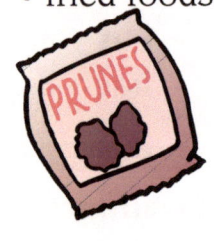
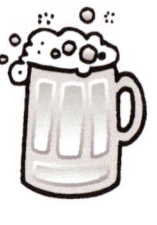

These foods may help if you become

It is important to have healthy stools (soft, formed stools which pass easily). You can have these by including plenty of liquids and fiber (after your colon has healed) in your diet. Fiber can be found in whole grain foods such as breads, brown and wild rice, beans and bran cereals. Exercising all or most days of the week will also help you have regular bowel movements. Brisk walking is a good exercise to do.

Sex

Like other parts of your life after colostomy surgery, getting back to sex can be exciting, as well as a bit scary. The surgery may affect your sex life, the ostomy will not. If you are still in pain or are not comfortable with the thought of having sex, don't. Sometimes your brain is ready before your body.

If you think you are ready, talk to your doctor or WOC nurse to make sure it's safe for you to have sex again. Many people can return to sex 4–6 weeks after surgery. For others, this is not nearly long enough. Everyone is different.

Once you've healed and the doctor says it's OK to have sex again, take it easy and go slowly. Sex may not be the same for a while.

Plan a time for sex when you feel good, and make it special and romantic. This can help you relax. The more relaxed you and your partner are, the more you will enjoy intimacy.

If you have any questions or concerns, talk with your doctor or WOC nurse.

If you're still not sure about having sex, talk to your partner. Share your feelings, fears and concerns. There are other ways you and your partner can find pleasure. If changing your usual routine is scary or makes either of you nervous, talk it over.

Once you're ready to have sex, these tips can help you and your partner enjoy it safely:

- Choose a time and place where you will be rested, relaxed and where you won't be interrupted.

- Keep your pouch empty and firmly adhered during sex. You can fold up the pouch and tape it to itself to make it smaller or use a security pouch.

- Some people with sigmoid colostomies can use a colostomy plug instead of a pouch. Ask your doctor or WOC nurse about this.

- Use a pouch cover, small piece of cloth or some type of lingerie to cover your pouch during sex if you'd like.

- Make sure your partner knows that sex won't hurt your stoma. It may bleed a few drops if it gets bumped, but that's OK.

- Find positions that are comfortable for you, and let your partner know about them.

- The United Ostomy Association (UOA) and American Cancer Society (ACS) publish booklets on the sexual aspects of living with an ostomy. For more information, see the inside back cover.

Helpful hints

- With your pouch in place, you can **shower or bathe as you did before** you had an ostomy. In the shower, **avoid spraying water directly on your pouch**. In the bath, avoid **letting the water come up over your pouch**.

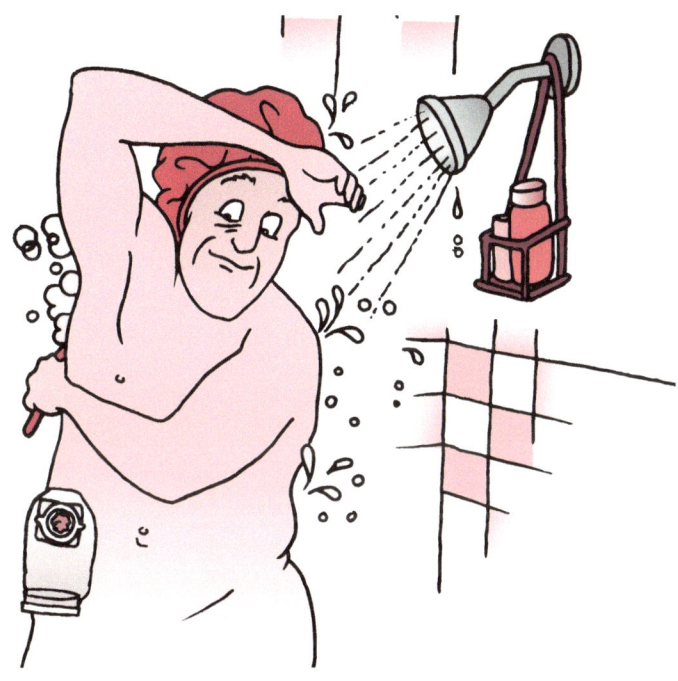

- **After changing your pouch, it is best to wait an hour before you shower**. But it is OK to shower, without your pouch.

- **Do not drive** a car until your doctor tells you it's OK.

- **Avoid heavy lifting** (5 pounds or more) **for 4–6 weeks** after surgery (1 gallon of milk weighs 5 pounds).

- **Rest between activities.**

- **Empty your pouch before you exercise.**

- If hair grows around the stoma, clip with scissors and dry shave with a razor on skin powdered with a skin barrier powder.

- Ostomy products are available in nearly every country in the world. But be prepared and **take your own supplies in your carry-on luggage when you travel**.

- When you travel, check with your WOC nurse to see if there is a WOC nurse where you are going. This is helpful if you have an emergency.

- **Put together an ostomy "emergency kit"** in case you have to change your pouch when you are away from home. Include:

  - an extra pouch

  - a new skin barrier wafer (or flange)

  - skin products (stoma powder, skin sealant, stoma paste)

  - plastic bags to put your old pouches in

  - an extra pouch clamp

  - paper towels

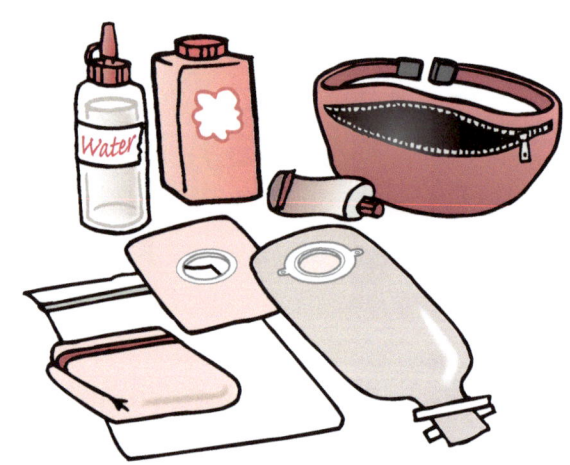

Women can use a cosmetic bag. Men can use a "fanny pack" or a travel kit to hold supplies.

Resources

These organizations may help you learn more about your colostomy. Ask about Support Groups that are in your area.

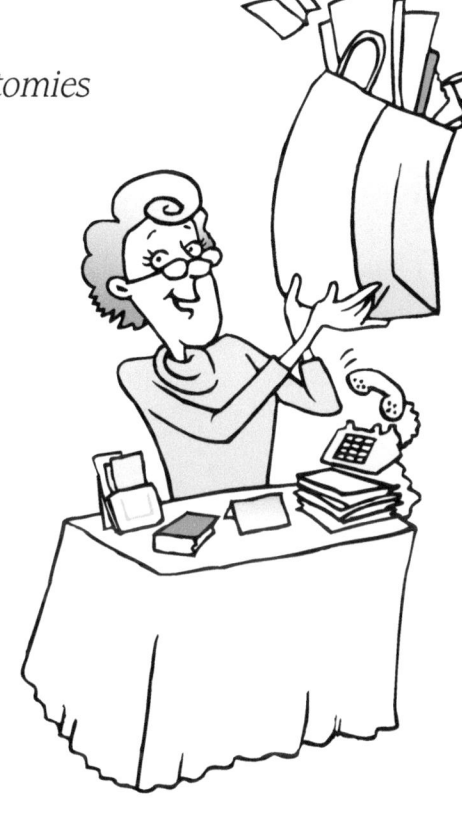

**United Ostomy Association
of America, Inc. (UOAA)**
An organization of people who have ostomies
P.O. Box 512
Northfield, MN 55057-0512
(800) 826-0826
www.ostomy.org

**Wound, Ostomy and
Continence Nurses Society**
*To find a WOC nurse in your area,
please visit the WOCN Society website
at wocn.org*

American Cancer Society (ACS)
(800) ACS-2345
cancer.org

Order this book from:

PRITCHETT & HULL ASSOCIATES, INC.
3440 OAKCLIFF RD NE STE 110
ATLANTA GA 30340-3006

1-800-241-4925

Published and distributed by:
Pritchett & Hull Associates, Inc.

Printed in the U.S.A.